22 Ideas:
Coping with Cancer

22 Ideas:
Coping with Cancer

*an inspirational guide
to surviving a cancer diagnosis
and thriving
as a cancer survivor*

by
Dalene Entenmann

"Yes to 22 ideas!"

Bernie Siegel, M.D., author of Love, Medicine &
Miracles and most recently
A Book of Miracles - Inspiring True Stories of
Healing, Gratitude and Love

*"Dalene Entenmann has written a wonderful
guide for anyone who has received that dreaded
diagnosis of "I'm afraid it's cancer."*

*And if I had my way, this guide would be given
to every patient at the moment the Oncologists
delivers that news."*

Patrick J. Murphy, co-author Heart Wide Open,
Self-Care for Caregivers

*"22 Ideas is a great companion to a challenging
journey. Uplifting and reassuring, it's like having
a good friend walk beside you."*

Sandi Kimmel, author and songwriter

*"Your 22 ideas are wonderful.
For well being and a good life,
I think everyone should read this,
cancer or not."*

Zachary S., reader review

Contents

Introduction 11
I Have Cancer 18
You Have Cancer 26

1. Faith in Your Healers 32
2. You Have Options 37
3. Be Your Own Advocate 42
4. Be Lifestyle Wise 46
5. Beware Quacks and Snake Oil Salesmen 53
6. Never Accept Blame 61
7. Rediscover Time, Reclaim Your Life 63
8. Start a Journal 66
9. Expressing Your Creative Self 70
10. Healing Power of Music 72
11. Healing Power of Laughter 76
12. Green Medicine 80
13. Fear In Small Doses 84
14. Plan for the Future 88
15. Forgiveness and Letting Go 91
16. You Are Not Alone 96
17. The Obligation in Giving Back 99
18. Write Love Letters 103
19. Create a Healing Shrine 106
20. Avoid Toxic People 108
21. Fill Your Life with Beauty 110
22. Expect to be a Survivor 114

You are Not Cancer 118
An Afterword --- Or Two 122
Resources 127

Introduction

Cancer does not occupy a space in my constellation of worry, until the day the surgeon says, "You have cancer." Up to this point, why isn't cancer a worry? Cancer happens to old people, and I am not old. Of course, this is a stereotypical notion about cancer for those who have yet to face cancer. Cancer can happen at any age, and does, from the young to the old and every age between.

One in two men and one in three women will face a cancer diagnosis in their lifetime. Their family and friends will be affected by the diagnosis. Eventually, given these statistics, who will not have a firsthand experience of cancer? Cancer runs in families, it does not run in mine. I discover later, cancer does run in my family, only no one talked about it, as it is a relation and generation or two removed.

And finally, in daily life, a person only has so much time to worry over life, and mine is consumed with the usual; work, bills, parenting skills, weather, rabbits stealing my garden strawberries, world peace and bad hair days. I have other every day worries, but you get the idea.

Cancer does not cross into my galaxy of daily worry before I find the lump in my breast, then cancer is my only worry. I have cancer. Next thought? Does this mean I am going to die soon?

After the initial shock, sadness, tears, fear and anger of my cancer diagnosis, a pragmatic and practical question settles in; Now what?

I have cancer. Now what? Not to put too dramatic a spin on it, but I instinctively feel the answer to this simple two-word yet immeasurably profound question has the potential to shape not only the quality of my life, but equally so, the quantity of my life. Both the quality and quantity of my life rest in the answer to this question. With singular focus and steely resolve, it is imperative I answer this question to the very best of my ability.

The answer to "Now what?" leads to more questions, opening the door to a world of questions about healing and the healed.

Why do some cancer patients survive and others do not; is spontaneous remission real and how does that work; are there research-based alternative therapies proven to help in healing; how genetically determined is cancer; do my thoughts and emotions influence my physical body; how much is diet and nutrition a factor; does the environment play a role; are there geographical regions and cultures of people who have a lower incidence of cancer and what lifestyle secrets might they hold; other than the known risks of smoking, obesity, poor diet and lack of exercise, are there less obvious lifestyle habits that lead to cancer? Is the exclusion of all other ancient and alternative systems of medicine in the traditional conventional course of treatment; surgery, radiation, chemotherapy, and chemoprevention drugs adequate for the best and successful outcome in treating cancer? Or will I stand a better chance of healing and being healed if multiple disciplines of medicine are sought?

Conventional medicine is marvelous in treating the immediate, the emergency. If I have a broken bone, I want to go to a medical facility where they can properly set it and prescribe antibiotics as needed. If I am in a car accident, I want first responders to speedily whisk me away by ambulance to the nearest trauma center where highly trained emergency room physicians, surgeons and surgical nurses will expertly care for my injuries. If I have a cancerous tumor, I want it surgically removed. The sooner, the better.

Where surgery and first line of defense drugs can solve a physical trauma or medical event, there is no better system of medical care available than Western medicine.

Alternative therapies prescriptive course, or what we often classify as eastern-based medicine, seek to treat the whole person where the mind, body and spirit are regarded as an interconnected whole. As effective as conventional medicine is in treating an immediate medical crisis, alternative therapy is equally effective at treating chronic long-term malady or illness.

Cancer falls into both categories of immediate medical crisis and long-term chronic disease. Finding a cancerous tumor is an immediate medical crisis. Surviving cancer long-term and avoiding cancer recurrence falls more into the chronic disease category.

Depending on who you ask, current conventional medicine is not nearly as successful in treating chronic conditions as older forms of medicine from the east or mind body alternative therapies.

To their credit, western medicine scientists are beginning to conduct research studies into alternative therapies. Some of these alternative therapies are proving valuable to the increased quality of life, and with additional research based studies, might well prove valuable to the quantity of life for cancer survivors.

Cancer centers across the country are beginning to offer integrative therapy; alternative treatments combined with conventional cancer treatment. But integrative therapy is not the universal norm, not yet, and largely nonexistent at the time of my cancer diagnosis in 2002.

I admit, for the majority of my life, I held a skeptical view of many alternative therapies. This area of healing modalities is rife with those of dubious intent; new age woo hucksters, charlatans, and opportunistic con men who seek to profit off the misfortune and fear of others.

My wary pragmatic opinion of alternative therapies takes a decided shift in perspective after my cancer diagnosis. While I am more open to ideas I readily dismissed before, my critical skepticism remains a companion to my new found interest into the effectiveness of alternative therapy. I want to live longer than the oncologist is suggesting I might.

When the oncology team predicts I have a 50 percent chance of living five more years, I am motivated to look beyond my previously held prejudice against alternative therapies. In the days, and months, and years to come, my perspective and opinion on a good number of things will change in regard to what alternative therapies mean for healing.

Before I could start my investigations into the diverse fields of alternative therapies and mind body medicine, my long held belief about living and dying and my less than enthusiastic response to the odds my oncologist is offering is challenged and changed after I share the less than positive 50 percent odds with a friend.

"At least you know you have a 50 percent chance of living five years. No one has given me odds I will live to see tomorrow."

Not the most empathetic reaction. I sit with this for a minute until I realize I can look at the odds from a much different perspective, and in doing so, I can relax. And in relaxing, I set up a much better personal environment for healing. It is glass half empty, glass half full. I can choose to focus on a possible five short years of life left, or I have a full five more years to live.

I am going to believe I will beat the odds. At the same time, if I only have five more years of life ahead of me, I want it to be the best and happiest five years of my life. I want to tie up loose ends and in a traditional way live out my bucket list. I do not want to leave this life with unfinished business, past or present, or unrealized dreams. I will settle debts and forgive debts, literally and metaphorically, of all kind.

My goal is to grow into the best possible version of myself before I go, and to give myself permission to live life completely on my own terms. I will build a legacy of worth in the time I am given. There is no surgery or drug for that; I will need to realize this path elsewhere.

In my quest to include as much hope and healing to the beginning days of cancer treatment and to the months, and gratefully to the years that follow, I begin research in earnest.

The 22 ideas I share in this book are not meant to stand as a substitute for conventional cancer treatments, I am not against these and I hold much hope in continuing research and new treatment discoveries. The ideas are an integrative approach meant to compliment; a gathering place at the crossroad where western medicine leaves off and alternative therapies begin.

And to introduce emerging and new ideas for health from scientists and cutting edge thinkers who suggest, based on advances in scientific understanding about how the basic structure of our universe works, and how we work within it, that the current healthcare paradigm of treatment needs a more expansive and inclusionary approach to reflect what science continues to discover.

Some of the new ideas, some of the unfamiliar philosophy, can be off-putting. It is easy to enter into the fields of body mind medicine and come away with the notion we are placing blame on the patient. If only you thought this; or felt this; or did this; you would not be ill. Let me be very clear about the reality of this misguided philosophy; at any point in time, we are all doing the best we can with what we know at the time.

I Have Cancer

"Most people live in a very restricted circle
of their potential being.
They make use of a very small portion
of their possible consciousness,
and of their soul's resources in general,
much like a man who, out of his whole bodily
organism, should get into the habit
of using and moving only his little finger.

Great emergencies and crises
show us how much greater
our vital resources are than we had supposed."

William James

I have cancer. In the first moments after being told I have cancer, my breath catches and pauses out of rhythm. I am terrorized by the diagnosis of a disease with no guaranteed positive outcomes. My loved ones are terrified for me. As hearts are dropping into a pool of sadness, no one is breathing deeply.

At the time of diagnosis, the odds given for surviving five years with my cancer, a metastasized invasive lobular breast cancer, is an even 50 percent split. Five years without a cancer recurrence is an invisible milestone upping the probabilities for long-term cancer survivorship beyond five years.

My odds do not inspire great confidence for reaching the five year mark. Hope, yes, same as a gambler hopes the bet he places will be the winning bet. But confidence? Not until the wheel stops spinning and the little bouncy ball settles into a slot of red or black, and depending on where I placed my bet, will I know if I win or lose.

For five long years, the roulette wheel spins, and spins, and spins, as the ever present uncertainty of cancer's return fills me with a constant daily dread.

At five years, I am still on this side of living and as far as tests reveal, still cancer free. The cancer specialists and statisticians who gave me a 50 percent chance of surviving cancer five years are half wrong. I am still here. The physician who silently gazed at me with pity when I proclaimed cancer will not be the death of me expressed a misdirected sympathy.

I. Am. Still. Here.

Now, according to statistics, the odds are more in my favor. The roulette wheel bouncy ball and I land on the right side of 50 percent. For now, I win.

From the fifth to sixth year of cancer survivorship, I find myself breathing deeper. During the first five years, every twinge, ache and pain heralds a potential warning of cancer returned. By the end of the sixth year of cancer survivorship, aches and pains are aches and pains. Transient in origin. Not a cataclysmic apocalyptic message from my body.

The seventh year of cancer survivorship is a true turning point. I rarely think about cancer. I certainly do not worry about cancer. By the seventh year, the memory of a cancer diagnosis begins to fade as simply one more historical fact in a life containing many historical facts.

On the celebration of my eighth year anniversary as a cancer survivor, I find the second lump. Two inches below my armpit, on the side of my ribcage. I hopefully reason the lump is a knotted muscle from overly enthusiastic spring gardening. To be on the safe side, I make an appointment to see our family physician.

"It appears to be a mass about the size of a golf ball deep in the muscle. Given your history, I think we need to send you to see a surgeon," suggests the furrow browed doctor.

This is not how I imagine the conversation before the office visit. My expectation is a prescriptive treatment for an innocuous malady of pulled muscle as typically recommended: ice pack, aspirin and time.

He does not need to say the word cancer as the possible concern. After all, we are both aware of my history.

Did I hear the roulette wheel stop spinning? Did I just watch the bouncy ball land on black when I bet on red?

In the first few moments, all initial thought and emotion I experienced during the first cancer diagnosis flood back as if I never advanced beyond that place and time. There is the familiar stunned shock, the inability to catch my breath, the anger, and foremost concern for my family.

As a mother, I spend my life as most mothers do; motherly protecting my children from what scares, both real and imaginary. Once again, as happened eight years before, I am the very circumstance I try to shield from my children. Cancer is forcing me to bring fear and an all consuming anxiety of foreboding doom into their lives. The guilt is overwhelming.

The surgeon diagnoses the lump as an enlarged lymph node and schedules surgery within the week. I say the cancer word out loud. In his trained medical opinion, does he think this is cancer?

His reply is the same as the family physician. "Given your history ..." and exits the exam room.

There are many new thoughts running through my mind in the days before this surgery and a potential diagnosis of cancer recurrence. Have I simply managed to overshoot the statistics predicting my death by three years? Has the physician's look of pity for what he believed to be my delusional proclamation of cancer not being the death of me lo those eight years ago been more accurate than my declared certainty of living a long life? Have all the organic, nutritional, physical, mental, and spiritual lifestyle choices in the last eight years been an act of futility?

I feel healthier and happier now than ever before, and yet, are the studies all wrong and the future is in fact determined simply on genetics? Does nothing we do make a difference? Are we left to the fickle and utterly random unfeeling fate of a spinning wheel and a bouncing ball and circumstances beyond our control?

The tumor is benign. Not cancer. Eight years ago, when I discover a lump in my breast, the physician waves it off, assuring me it is symptomatic of any number of minimally worrisome medical problems. He is wrong. The lump is an aggressive cancer. Eight years later, the physician and surgeon are not certain it is any number of simple transitory medical issues, given my history.

This time the lump is not cancer. I feel a need to repeat this often before the reality sinks in and I am free to deeply breathe again a second time. Perhaps I did do something, making informed health and lifestyle choices from the first cancer diagnosis to this benign tumor, which did affect the outcome from life threatening to more than just a lucky break. Who knows.

The cancer recurrence scare shapes my fearful anxiety consuming thoughts and feelings regarding cancer different from the first diagnosis of cancer. Am I currently as angst ridden and terrified of a cancer recurrence as I felt before facing an actual second time around cancer scare? No, because I know if cancer returns I will face the cancer head on and do whatever I need to do for the best possible outcome. Before the cancer scare I am consumed with fear at the mere possibility of a cancer recurrence. Actually experiencing a second cancer scare is not as frightening as imagined. With that, the daily haunting of the shadowy presence of a cancer threat lingering in my daily consciousness evaporates in the misty recesses of my mind.

Most importantly, time and experience taught me this: cancer does not automatically equal death. I realize it is difficult to talk someone out of their fears, especially if those fears are based on the reality of a previous experience, but I am going to try to talk you out of it. Should you be faced with a second cancer scare or actual cancer recurrence, know that one, it will not be as scary as you imagine beforehand and two, if you overcame cancer once, believe you can do it again.

I am not a doctor or cancer researcher or spiritual adviser. I am a cancer survivor. I am not certain which actions I took or decisions I made for my mental, emotional and spiritual wellness keep me living longer than statisticians predict at the time of my cancer diagnosis.

Or if I am still here by sheer blind luck and a gambler's good fortune. Either way, the quality of my life in the last ten years is measurably better on all levels, and that alone is a reason to share what I learned.

For clarity, I do want to state I believe optimum healing often rests at the intersection of traditional western medicine, research based eastern alternative therapies and liberally applied common sense. In my opinion, both disciplines and a no-nonsense perspective have their place and value in health and wellness.

Perhaps something in my story and in sharing ideas learned from surviving a cancer diagnosis to thriving as a cancer survivor will matter, that if you know, will help you in surviving a cancer diagnosis and thriving as a cancer survivor too.

In the 22 Ideas: Coping With Cancer guide, you will be offered ideas to help shape, define and design your own healing path, as well as inspiring quotes and relevant personal entries from my journal.

At the end of the guide are online resources with website addresses which allow you to learn more about the ideas of interest to you. There is no one path to healing.

You Have Cancer

*"An angel can illumine the thought and mind
by strengthening the power of vision
and by bringing within reach truth
which the angel contemplates."*

St. Thomas Aquinas

Those three words are a time stopping life changing breath catching punch in the gut. I know. I know how you feel. I know what you are thinking. I have occupied the place and time you find yourself today.

All at once, life ceases holding the limitless potential of possibilities. Where most of us take for granted the expansive idea of a plentiful future in a life measured by multiple more decades to come, days no longer stretch into guaranteed years before us.

No, at the moment, there seem to be more yesterdays than there might be tomorrows.

From the core of being, the safe connection of time to life is shattered and scattered and tossed up in the air by an arbitrarily impersonal faceless fate. Logically, we are aware immortality does not exist, and yet, we conduct our lives as if there is a thread of immortality to our existence here on earth.

When busy living, few give thought to disease or death. When the center of our focus turns to the true nature of mortality, we react with shock and dismay. Even if we are peacefully reconciled to the reality that our time is limited on this planet, we certainly do not want cancer to be the cause for our exit. These realities are almost too large to embrace.

Suddenly threatened with the untimely inevitable, and any illusion of a life stretching on into old age, we panic more than a bit inside.

The weight of emotions from the shift in awareness from immortality to the fragility of life is crushing. While we are attempting to process a swirl of disbelief, fear, anger, and sadness, we are presented with the best options to treat our specific cancer.

Oh yes, while we are falling apart inside, we need to keep our wits about us. There are choices to consider and decisions to be made. The task is monumental.

Let me take a moment to tell you, while you might not have all the time in the world, you do have time to take a moment, take a deep breath, and find a calm inner balance before making final decisions.

Whatever lay before you in the days to come, coming at it from the calm center of your being is optimally your best bet.

After a treatment plan is agreed upon, there is nothing more to do other than show up at the hospital, cancer clinic, and oncologist office at the specified times for treatment and wait for the test results of each treatment to determine the success of treatment.

Surgeons, physicians, technicians and oncologists take care of our physical being. Our mental, emotional and spiritual wellness are ours to tend.

I have been told I have cancer.

You are being told you have cancer.

Now what? For now, remember to breathe.

In daily life, minor events can cause anxiety and stress. Major life events can cause overwhelming anxiety and stress. A recent cancer diagnosis is a major event. Long-term cancer survivors can suffer from chronic anxiety and stress, as worry over cancer recurrence can persist for years. Minor, major or chronic anxiety and stress are counterproductive in achieving and maintaining good health.

The conversation, between someone I meet who is recently diagnosed with cancer to long-term survivors who cannot shake the fear of a cancer recurrence, varies depending on specific circumstance. Our visit always ends with the same advice. At first, remember to breathe.

Our breathing is so automatic, we forget, or never realize, there is more than one way to breathe. Breathing allows us to live, mastering our breath allows us to live well. If someone is suffering from anxiety or stress, they are breathing shallow. Shallow breathing is not breathing well.

Shallow breathing causes the chest to expand. Deep breathing causes the chest and abdomen to expand. To take a deep breath, slowly inhale through the nose, expanding the abdomen first, followed by the expansion of the chest. As you slowly exhale, either through the nose or mouth, allow the abdomen to fall, followed by chest.

Choose comfortable clothing and position. A beginning technique in learning to breathe well involves lying down, with one hand on abdomen and one hand on chest. This allows you to feel the rise and fall of both abdomen and chest with each inhalation and exhalation of breath.

As you slowly inhale and exhale, focus on the sound of your breath. If the mind wanders, or unwelcome anxious or stressful thoughts filter in, return your focus to the sound of breathing.

According the National Center for Complementary and Alternative Medicine,

"People may use relaxation techniques as part of a comprehensive plan to treat, prevent, or reduce symptoms of a variety of conditions including stress, high blood pressure, chronic pain, insomnia, depression, labor pain, headache, cardiovascular disease, anxiety, chemotherapy side effects, and others."

According to the 2007 National Health Interview Survey, which included a comprehensive survey of complementary and alternative medicine use by Americans, currently 12.7 percent of American adults use deep breathing exercises.

Relaxation is more than a state of mind; it physically changes the way your body functions. When your body is relaxed breathing slows, blood pressure and oxygen consumption decrease, and some people report an increased sense of well-being.

For now, remember to breathe.

Deeply.

Slowly.

Then consider your choices.

Then make your decisions.

Then have faith in your healers,

and faith in yourself.

1

Faith in Your Healers

*"Let me not pray to be sheltered from dangers
but to be fearless in facing them.*

*Let me not beg for the stilling of my pain
but for the heart to conquer it.*

*Let me not crave in anxious fear to be saved
but hope for the patience to win my freedom."*

Tagore

Physicians are people with the same strengths and weaknesses as every other human on the planet. Some are as intimidated and terrified of cancer as the patient. These are not the healers for you. Regardless of diagnosis, staging or statistical probabilities, who wants a doctor who believes cancer is an automatic death sentence? Or even a highly probable death? Not me. Not you.

The most appalling story I hear involves a woman I have not met. She finds a lump in her breast and visits a doctor. During the exam, before a biopsy is performed or staging determined, she is told she has six months to live. When I am told this, I ask that a message be passed on to her. In no uncertain terms, I suggest she seek a second opinion and never return to this doctor's office again.

I have a great respect for doctors, but they are not gods. They do not possess clairvoyant powers. No one can say with complete authority someone is going to die in six months. Any doctor might share statistics, a great doctor will share statistics and say immediately after, "yes, but those are only general statistics – everyone is different". A doctor who will say you are going to die in a certain window of time? Run from them as fast as you can. Yes, she got a second opinion, and years after that horrendous first doctor visit, she is still living today.

In the early weeks after a cancer diagnosis, there is a dizzying array of doctors to meet, each with their own specialty. I devise a simple litmus test to determine who I want on my medical team. During initial consultations, I state with absolute certainty "cancer is not going to kill me."

Do I believe this statement with absolute certainty? I want to, but no, not absolutely. Tiny doubts dance in the background of my proclamation.

However, I do want everyone on my medical team to operate from an optimistic belief in my longevity. They might not truly believe with absolute certainty in my long term survival, but I need them to convincingly convey the belief my survival is not only possible, but highly probable.

When I say "cancer is not going to kill me," I focus on immediate reaction and facial expression. If I sense doubt or pity, I cross the doctor off my list of potential team players. Your litmus test might not be mine, but you need to devise one before you meet with any medical professional to sort out who you choose for your team. With cancer, we might get one chance to do it right.

Look for compassion, those who take the time to listen, those who make time to answer your questions. When you meet with them, feel in your heart what your intuition is telling you. If you do not believe in your healers, keep looking until you find healers you can believe in.

Then have faith they will do everything they can, as expertly as they can, to help you survive cancer. Let them know you will be doing everything you can to help yourself survive, while they are doing everything they can to help you survive a cancer diagnosis and live beyond this disease as a cancer survivor.

May 2002

Dear Cancer Diary,

The radiologist is blunt but not unkind in her honesty. This is cancer and the cancer does not look good. She is quick to add an element of hope. Effective treatments are available. Then with a caveat she cautiously adds to her assurance of hope, until the biopsy is performed, no one can know exactly what the cancer cells are doing and the path they will most likely take in the days ahead. Basically, at this moment, what I have in knowledge, is the following:

This is cancer.
The cancer is aggressive.
There are treatments available for this cancer.

How effective depends on the next round of tests.

In other words, depending on factors still unknown, the cancer might or might not be effectively treatable. I will not know how much of a battle I will need to engage in with this cancer, to win the rest of my life from a disease designed to take life from me, until the bone scan, chest xray and biopsy provide a working blueprint of the adversarial activity going on within my body.

Regardless of outcome, my life will never be the same. I am in a war I did not volunteer for and will need to learn what it truly means to be a warrior.

On May 7th, 2002, I drive home in contemplation and concern for my children. I am sitting in my parked car in the driveway and imagining I can stare through the walls of our home. My family is inside. In the next ten minutes I will deliver news that will change everyone's life. How can I avoid the unavoidable shattering of innocence in their world? How to protect them from their own fear and pain?

This day is a week before Mother's Day, less than two weeks before my birthday. My children are still young but old enough to be frightened by cancer. Will I have the courage and resolve to conquer my own fear and pain? Will I be able to carry my children and myself through the battlefields with dignity and strength, and not lose heart along the way?

2

You Have Options

*"Knowing others is intelligence
knowing yourself is true wisdom
Mastering others is strength
mastering yourself is true power"*

Lao-Tzu

*"Make friends with the angels, who though
invisible are always with you. Often invoke
them, constantly praise them, and make good
use of their help and assistance in all your
temporal and spiritual affairs."*

Saint Francis de Sales

You might not like most of your options, but you have options. A one-size-fits-all treatment approach of throwing everything at the wall in hope something sticks is quickly becoming a thing of cancer treatment past.

Each cancer treatment brings with it a statistical probability in cancer survival. Each cancer treatment side effects, both short term and long term, might alter the quality of life years after treatment. All the positives of each individual treatment need to be weighed against all the negatives in deciding which calculated risks are worth taking, and you have the power to make the final decisions.

In the beginning, the choices in different courses of treatment available and the decisions you need to make can feel as if you are in information overload, and your feeling won't be far wrong. Take it one step at a time. Keep a notebook. Take notes. Write down questions that come to mind before and after each meeting.

Is the oncologist recommending a take it slow or more aggressive treatment approach? Will you opt for a port or take a chance on vein collapse during chemotherapy? Will you choose chemotherapy? Will you choose radiation treatment? If there is surgery, will you need the reconstruction services of a plastic surgeon? Is hormone drug treatment of benefit in treating your specific cancer? Are targeted treatments offered? Depending on the staging of your cancer, are clinical trials an option? If you are of childbearing age, what steps in preserving your fertility do you need to take before treatment begins?

Does the cancer clinic offer social services and psychologists on staff? Are there nutritionists, physical therapists and exercise programs? Do they practice any form of complementary medicine or do they offer a network for integrative therapies? Do they offer a list of online resources and local community support groups?

Do you have choices between drugs and treatments? Will your medical cancer team allow you to make a choice? If not, why not? There might be a plausible reason, but you need to clearly understand the reason for any lack of choice.

Take your time. You do not have all the time in the world, but you have time to research the recommended options. Absolutely, get a second opinion. When you are certain which cancer treatments are the right ones for you, then and only then, consent to treatment. Do not allow yourself to feel you have no choices. Of course you do, every step of the way.

June 2002

Dear Diary,

The biopsy is only the beginning. The surgeon calls to explain the biopsy reading indicates an invasive lobular cancer. Surgical removal of the tumor and lymph nodes will determine the margin and spread of the cancer. At the time of his call, if he said more, I do not hear him.

Time stops. The road ends. Standing on the stage of my life, I hear the final curtain call with one word: cancer. Without further doubt or last minute reprieve, I have cancer. All hope is dashed my brush with mortality is a near miss and not the full on collision with the idea of death.

I listen for my own breathing because I wonder if I am breathing. The awareness of breath is all the height of attention I can bring to this moment in time, and the width of vision I can realistically allow myself. Where do I go from here? Will there be any here to there? What is my next step? Does it matter what I do?

Yes, it matters. I matter. My life matters.

I am surviving my first minute after the last minute of the life that ends so abruptly with one word: cancer.

I am, in this first next minute, and the next minute after that, surviving cancer. I am a cancer survivor. I will need to remember, remind myself, from minute to minute, in the minutes of days to come.

I am and will be a cancer survivor.

"Be at peace with your own soul,
then heaven and earth
will be at peace with you.

Enter eagerly into the treasure house
that is within you,
you will see the things that are in heaven;

for there is but one single entry to them both.

The ladder that leads to the Kingdom
is hidden within your soul,
and in your soul you will discover
the stairs by which to ascend."

Saint Issac

3

Be Your Own Advocate

Come to the edge.
"We can't. We're afraid."
"Come to the edge."
"We can't. We will fall!"
"Come to the edge."
And they came.
And he pushed them.
And they flew.

Guillaume Apollinaire

"Hope is the pillar that holds up the world.
Hope is the dream of a waking man."

Pliny the Elder

The surgeon, the oncologist, the radiologist, the chemotherapy nurse, the plastic surgeon, the oncology social worker, all the medical professionals and health care workers are trained to do the jobs they do. Most likely you are not trained in any of these specialties. It can be impressive what they know and what they can accomplish. At the same time, do not feel you are in a position of powerlessness because you do not have matching educational credentials.

From the start, actively participate in your own care. You have a right and responsibility to know the how, what, where, when and why of agreed upon cancer treatments. Ask questions until there is no doubt in your understanding and continue to ask questions as you move through treatment phases. Speak up when something does not feel right or when you need a clearer understanding about a procedure or treatment.

Do not be afraid or intimidated to bring information you have found of interest and ask their opinion. With the internet, access to new information, new research studies, and new treatments are published on a consistent basis, and easy to find. However, as everyone knows, just because it's on the internet, does not make it valid or worthwhile.

Asking for an opinion and insight from a medical

professional cannot hurt. At the very least, you will be able to add their perspective to your own.

Expect the medical professionals you meet during cancer treatment to stop and take time to address any and all concerns.

While being timid and quiet and never speaking up is not recommended, conversely, take into consideration your medical team has many other patients in their care.

Buy yourself a journal dedicated to your appointments and treatments. No one ever thinks they are going to forget such important events or conversations, but we can. To be on the safe side, consider bringing a family member or friend with you. They might well remember something you forget afterward. Or tape the conversation, to be played back when you are in a more comfortable setting.

Before each visit, write your questions down as they come to you between visits. It is amazing how many important questions I had, when sitting in the exam room or treatment room, escaped my memory.

Only returning home did I remember what I wanted to ask. Not only that, but if you have written questions, it helps your doctor or nurse with their time management, as they can address each one in a timely logical sequence.

If you have found new research studies or information relating to various treatments, print out what you find and ask the doctor if he or she can look it over and give you his or her opinion. They might be able to do it at the time of your appointment, or later when they have a moment to spare.

Create a file folder for your research.

In being your own advocate, expect respect, extend respect, and speak up. After all, this is your one life, as you, now.

4

Be Lifestyle Wise

*"I tell you the truth,
if you have faith as small as a mustard seed,
you can say to this mountain,
'Move from here to there'
and it will move."*

Jesus

*"Fear knocked at the door.
Faith answered.
No one was there."*

Increasing evidence suggests, and many leading cancer experts, cancer research institutions and cancer organizations are concluding, lifestyle choices are risk factors for as much as 30 to 50 percent of cancer occurrence.

Lifestyle choices are in our control. What we eat, where we live, personal habits and our involvement in physical activity are all lifestyle choices.

Some cancer patients eliminate all processed food and begin cooking from scratch; selecting only fresh, local and organic vegetables, fruits and limited portions of meat; or eliminate meat completely for a plant-based diet; or choose to create meals following the low glycemic index; or follow a macrobiotic diet.

Other cancer patients will take stock of where they live and decide they eventually need to live in a place with cleaner air, cleaner water and a cleaner environment.

Still others will join a gym, begin a daily walking habit or take a yoga class.

Research each of these diets, experiment, and find the one most realistic for you. Same holds true in where you live and choices in physical activities. Rather than seeing the change in lifestyle habits as deprivation in what you might be giving up or a chore in one more thing to add to your already too many things to do life, embrace it as an opportunity to discover a new style of life and a wonderful new way of living that is better for your health.

If you are uncomfortable or have concerns with changes and making the healthiest choices for your individual health, consult with a registered dietitian, certified nutritionist or physical therapist. For additional help or guidance, many cancer clinics are happy to refer you to reputable practitioners. If not, cancer community members will step up and share what they know works for them.

The Mediterranean Diet, considered one of the healthiest diets on the planet and the easiest to transition into, is primarily a plant-based diet.

According to the Mediterranean Diet Pyramid, vegetables, fruits, whole grains, beans, nuts, legumes, seeds, olive oil, herbs and spices are consumed daily. Fish and seafood are consumed at least two times a week. Poultry, eggs, cheese and yogurt are consumed weekly. Meats and sweets are consumed once or twice a month.

A Vegetarian Diet is a plant-based diet that does not include meat, poultry or fish. Lacto-ovo vegetarians include dairy and eggs while a lacto-vegetarian will include dairy but not eggs.

According to the Vegetarian Diet Pyramid, include whole grains, bread, rice and pasta liberally; vegetables and fruits generously; dairy, legumes and meat alternatives (tofu, tempeh, seitan) moderately and fats, healthy fats like coconut and olive oil, and sweets and salt sparingly.

For hormonal driven cancers, there is some controversy over soy's potential effect on estrogen. To be on the safe side, if your cancer is affected by hormone levels and it is a concern, simply eliminate soy-based products. On a vegetarian diet, there are satisfying protein alternatives to soy.

As research continues to indicate, animal fats and protein can raise your risk for cancer, as well as a number of other diseases, and in general shorten your lifespan.

The health advantage of a vegetarian diet is currently making it a more attractive mainstream choice. With balance and planning, a vegetarian diet can meet the complete nutritional needs for all of any age.

A Vegan Diet follows the same diet pyramid as vegetarians, only vegans do not consume any dairy or animal food products, including eggs and honey. At first, this diet choice might seem the most difficult to adopt as it appears strict in practice. However, if you stop and take a look at the typical westernized meat and potatoes diet, you will find many side dishes are already vegetarian or vegan.

Vegans do need to supplement their meatless dairy-free diet with several nutrients lacking in sufficient quantity like iron and vitamin b12. This is fairly easy to accomplish. The general advice is to follow a vegetarian diet first, and transition to veganism after the vegetarian diet becomes familiar and comfortable.

A Glycemic Index Diet focuses on carbohydrates. Carbohydrates are simple and complex sugars and starches. All carbohydrates are not the same. Some carbohydrates cause a sharp spike in blood glucose, while others help to maintain a steady blood sugar level. Low glycemic foods are preferable to high glycemic foods. To follow a low Glycemic Index Diet is to choose carbohydrate foods based on the food's effect on blood sugar levels.

The Glycemic Food Index is divided in three categories: low <55, medium <70 and high for any food with a rating over 70. Using the Glycemic Food Index chart, carbohydrate foods are listed from low to high. Most vegetables rank as the lowest in glycemic load, followed by some fruits, whole grains and legumes. You need to be careful. While asparagus ranks at 14, potato ranks at 85. While cherries rank at 22 and peaches at 42, watermelon ranks at 72. The Glycemic Index Charts are readily available on the internet.

To date, there is conflicting evidence about the role of blood sugar levels to cancer risk. Glucose affects us on a cellular level, so it stands to reason making the best choices of food with the lowest glycemic load is the most beneficial to overall health. Traditionally, this diet is associated with weight loss, which is a plus in long term cancer prevention.

A Macrobiotic Diet is more than a diet; it is a philosophy and way of life in relation to food. Although the following percentages can vary by region, the Americanized version of the macrobiotic diet recommends a daily intake of food that includes 50 to 60 percent whole grains, 20 to 30 percent vegetables and fruits, 5 to 10 percent beans, 5 to 20 percent fish, nuts, seeds, seaweed and miso; and include two cups of soup a day.

The emphasis is on locally grown food. Fruits are allowed as long as they grow in the area you live. All food is judged by yin and yang qualities. Yin food is defined as having cold and light characteristics and yang for hot and heavy characteristics. Certain vegetables are not advised as too extreme in yin or yang, for example: avocados, beets, eggplant, peppers, potatoes, spinach and tomatoes. Brown rice is considered a perfect balance of yin and yang. There are rules to the types of utensils and methods of cooking food. Lastly, food is to be eaten slowly and chewed thoroughly.

Just as important as what you eat and the diet you adopt is how you eat and where you sit down to eat. Enjoy mealtime in the company of family and friends. Afterward, take a walk. Exercise is an equally important lifestyle choice in cancer prevention.

On the subject of exercise. Not a gym rat? Never run a marathon? Have no desire to join a gym or lace up a pair of running shoes?

Guess what? One of the healthiest forms of exercise is walking. If need be, start with a short stroll and work up to brisk walking, each day adding a few more minutes to your walk. Brisk walking at least 30 minutes a day is a terrific means of exercise. Grab a friend or family member and make your walk a standing date. Later, if you feel inclined, you might give weight bearing exercises a try.

The point is to move. Find a fun way to accomplish this, and call it exercise. In addition, take a few breaks in your day to meditate and breath deeply.

5

Beware

Quacks

&

Snake Oil Salesmen

Sad but true, the unscrupulous loiter in the shadows to take advantage of the vulnerable and frightened.

The most common spiel begins from a premise of conspiracy. The government, the scientists, the pharmaceutical companies are all in cahoots and collectively blocking, suppressing, or preventing public knowledge of a cancer cure. Primarily, the reasoning goes, they cannot make a profit from known cures.

A hidden cure for cancer the quack or snake oil salesman is only too happy to reveal to you or treat you with - for a princely price of course. Ironic. Apply the smallest amount of common sense street smarts, and here is where the conspiracy theory falls apart.

During our lifetime, one in two men and one in three women will be diagnosed with cancer. Stands to reason the government officials, scientists and pharmaceutical employees, accused of hiding a cancer cure from the rest of the world, are touched by cancer. With those odds, during the arc of a lifetime, they will face a diagnosis of cancer or someone they love will face a diagnosis of cancer. Who in their right mind believes they will stand by and allow themselves, their loved ones or the neighbor down the street, to suffer needlessly if there is indeed an existing cancer cure?

This is not to suggest government officials, scientists and pharmaceutical employees are all pure in intent. No, some government officials make promises to large campaign donors that do not serve the public interest, some scientists who run research studies can be influenced by the entities funding the research and some pharmaceutical company employees are rewarded for the bottom line profit they make the pharmaceutical company, and care about little else.

Most often, those who work for the lesser good are found out and exposed by their contemporaries who work for the greater good. Or by an expose penned by an intrepid investigative reporter. The misguided, less well intended or nefarious wolf in sheep clothing cannot stay hidden forever.

Only the most jaded among us can believe, as a whole, the world is filled with anything other than good people who mean well and will gladly help in any way possible to alleviate suffering.

Yes, be skeptical, cynical and cautious - of the very group who encourages skepticism and cynicism - quacks and snake oil salesmen.

At the same time, do not dismiss out of hand many millennium of mind, body and energy healing traditions like acupuncture, yoga, aromatherapy, massage, meditation, prayer, talk therapy and visualization without first researching what these healing modalities might offer.

Some of the benefits from these alternative therapies can contribute to stress and anxiety reduction, boost the immune function, increase physical flexibility after surgery, lessen nausea during chemotherapy, promote a greater sense of spiritual connection and psychologically strengthen a newly defined post cancer sense of self.

Even then, be wary of any program or any person who seeks to separate you from any substantial amount of money. Research into any of the aforementioned are easily investigated without financial cost or participated in with a minimal amount of investment.

Inquiry, research or a trial run in alternative therapies is reasonable, as long as you let your medical team know what you are doing before you begin.

Not every tradition or practice will offer the same benefit to every cancer patient. If you find an alternative healing practice that feels good and seems to offer benefit, consider integrating it into your conventional medical treatments.

Most people are familiar with prayer, talk therapy or support groups and have experienced the benefit of one or all three at some point in their life.

Following is an overview of a few of the therapies you might not be as familiar with in terms of complementary alternative treatments:

Acupuncture: Dating back thousands of years and associated with Traditional Chinese Medicine (TCM), an acupuncturist treats patients with ultra thin needles in an effort to manipulate meridian channels and balance the flow of energy in the body. Research indicates acupuncture is effective for nausea and pain.

Aromatherapy: Aromatherapy is the therapeutic use of essential oils from flowers, herbs, or trees. When inhaled, the use of essential oils have either a sedating or stimulating effect on the limbic system, or emotional center of our brain. Studies have shown benefit for mental, physical, emotional, and spiritual wellness. Aromatherapy can improve immune function, as well as reduce stress and anxiety.

Ayurvedic Medicine: This ancient (over 3,000 years old) medical practice focuses on the connection between body, mind and spirit. Treatments are tailored to the unique constitution of the individual and doshas: Vata, Pitta, and Kapha.

Energy therapy: Used to manipulate a body's energy fields, some energy therapies include Energy Medicine, Reiki, Therapeutic Touch, Healing Touch, Tai Chi and Qi Gong.

Massage therapy: A good massage can reduce stress and pain, lower blood pressure, improve circulation, dramatically relax the patient and aid in achieving an overall sense of well-being.

Meditation/Guided Meditation: The practice of meditation leads to a calm mind and reduction in stress, anxiety, fear and worry. Respected and well known practitioners in guided meditation are Brian Weiss, Jon Kabat-Zinn and Belleruth Naparstek. All three have published guided meditation videos on YouTube. You can find their work on many websites. After you decide which one resonates with you the most, you can purchase CDs, MP3s and books. Or check your library.

Supplements and Herbs: Supplements and herbal preparations are regulated, but not as strictly as other drugs. Responsibility for the most part is left to the manufacturers. In certain cases, when independent testing has been done, actual amounts of ingredients varied from label and in some instances, toxic substances were detected. To date, research based studies indicate a handful of supplements do show benefit. Two are vitamin D and if there is bone loss, calcium. And some supplements and herbs, combined with other medications, can lead to adverse effects.

Based on thousands of studies, hundreds of experts and an independent panel of scientists, the American Institute of Cancer Research and the World Cancer Research Fund do not recommend the use of supplements for cancer prevention.

A balanced whole foods diet rich in vegetables, fruits, grains, nuts and legumes, with minimal meat and dairy consumption, should provide all the nutrients required to maintain optimal health. With the exception of vitamin D.

Visualization/Guided Imagery: Creating mental images in your mind to reduce stress and promote relaxation, allowing the body an enhanced opportunity to heal, can be done on your own or with the aid of a guided imagery therapist. You can find different techniques and practitioners online, much the same as you will for guided meditation. With practice, guided imagery is highly effective. Athletes routinely use guided imagery to imagine crossing a finish line before beginning the race or prevailing against an opponent in competitive sport.

Yoga: The origins of yoga are rooted in an ancient Indian spiritual philosophy. Today, yoga is considered by many in the West as another form of exercise. Yoga offers health benefits through a combination of breathing techniques, meditation and physical postures. There are numerous styles of yoga offered, and if you are unfamiliar with yoga, ask friends, look for online recommendations, or get a referral from your healthcare provider or clinic.

If you are interested in exploring alternative and complementary therapies mentioned here and many others that are not, a good place to start is the National Center for Complementary and Alternative Medicine.

Again, for your own safety, and since you are working as a team, speak with your physician about any alternative therapies you are interested in or considering adding to your conventional treatments.

You might be surprised at the adverse effects some alternative treatments can have when combined with your conventional treatments.

6

Never Accept Blame

"We are here to do;
and through doing to learn;
and through learning to know;
and through knowing to experience wonder;
and through wonder to attain wisdom;
and through wisdom to find simplicity;
and through simplicity to give attention;
and through attention to see
what needs to be done."

Pirke Avot

"We do the best we can with what we know, and
when we know better, we do better."

Maya Angelou

Do not blame yourself or allow others to suggest that you caused your cancer. Accept responsibility for the lifestyle changes you can make to help with your healing now, but I repeat, never accept blame from yourself or others for a cancer diagnosis. Not only is this cruel and unwarranted but highly counter productive to healing.

Illness is not a punishment. Throughout history, very good people get sick, and very bad people can live a very long time. There are mysteries in this life, and who gets sick and who does not is one of those oft times unexplainable and illogical events having nothing at all to do with reward or punishment.

Cancer is not payback from the universe because you were in some way an awful person living a life full of wrongheaded choices or dastardly deeds. There is no karmic debt collector come calling. Exceptionally nice, giving and good people are diagnosed with cancer.

In addition, cancer did not happen to you because you developed a cluster of personality traits making you susceptible to cancer. Own any positive changes you might feel are worth taking in living a healthier life for mind, body and spirit, but do not own blame. Again, disease is not a judicious reward and punishment system.

7

Rediscover Time

Reclaim Your Life

*The secret of health for both mind and body
is not to mourn for the past, not to worry
about the future, or not to anticipate troubles,
but to live in the present moment
wisely and earnestly."*

Buddha

We live hurried hectic lives. We work too many hours. We schedule too many events. We spend an enormous amount of time getting from one place to the next as fast as possible. Why? What is driving us? And what are we missing along the way?

For one thing, we cannot be present or feel our feelings with any depth of understanding. There is no time to connect to ourselves, to others, or to life in meaningful ways.

In our minds, we live in the past, we live in the future, we are not present in the here and now. We lose so much now time. Yesterday does not truly exist, although we can keep experiencing it by remembering it over and over. The problem with that, is the memories we keep reliving are rarely good ones, and even if there are, they are not what is happening now. Tomorrow never comes. It is always today. It is always now. Stay here in the now.

Slow down. Eliminate the unnecessary. Unplug. Find ways to be in the present moment. You have important things to do in slowing down and refocusing, namely reconnecting with yourself and the very essence of your life.

What would you do if you had more time? Go to the spa? Take long walks? Lay on a grassy hillside and look for shapes in the clouds? Spend more time with family and friends? Lounge in a hammock and read from your favorite list of books? Write the Great American Novel? Paint the next masterpiece? Take a trip to a favorite destination? Invent a better mousetrap? Do good works in making this world a better place?

Choose to spend time in ways that make you feel good, that give you a sense of awe, meaning, renewal and enthusiasm for life.

You might need to sit down and spend some time contemplating and writing out a list of your personal priorities, the less obvious ones but equally important ones, of long lost interests, dreams and goals. Being busy, and living a hectic life, separates us from ourselves. This happens incrementally over time, so we are not aware of the separation to self. At first, we might not remember what our dreams are, what our heart longs for, what makes us feel good.

Simply eliminate the extraneous activities from the essential. The point is, the time is now. The time has always been now. The only permission you need is your own. Do not wait to give yourself permission to take the time to live your best possible life.

Rediscover your time. Reclaim your life.

8

Start a Journal

"Yesterday is a dream,
tomorrow but a vision.
But today well lived makes yesterday
a dream of happiness,
and every tomorrow
a vision of hope.
Look well, therefore, to this day."

Sanskrit Proverb

There are a variety of journals you can choose to write: some are pure fun, some lead to self understanding and growth, and all, in one way or the other, are healing. Well documented research indicates writing out thoughts and feelings in the pages of a journal provides positive therapeutic value. Psychologically, keeping a journal reduces anxiety and depression, two maladies a new cancer patient is likely to confront and continue to struggle with in the long term survivorship phase. Physically, journaling is shown to reduce stress and improve overall immune function.

Both our thoughts and feelings, especially the disquieting ones, go undetected or get trapped in a mobius strip on a never ending muddled loop if left unexpressed beyond our deeper inner self.

After a time, distressing thoughts and feelings can create a distorted view of possibility and potential for positive outcomes, often making worry more worrisome, stress more stressful and hope seemingly impossible to hold. These thoughts and emotions can also take an unhealthy toll on the physical body.

For your own mental and emotional health, journaling allows you the ability to say out loud in written form what you are thinking and feeling. Keeping a journal moves these thoughts and feelings into the external world allowing for a clarity of perspective, a clearing of thoughts and emotions you might not want to hang onto, which in turn increases overall well being.

Journaling is a safe, non-judgmental avenue for self expression. Unless you want to share your journal, your writing is private.

The type of journal you keep depends on your interests. Some types of journals and styles of writing will appeal to one person and not the other. To begin, here is a starting point for some of the different journals you might like to try:

1. Morning Pages: Julie Cameron, author of The Artist's Way, started this practice. When you wake, start writing. Do not edit yourself or think too much about what you are writing. Simply start writing in a stream of consciousness, and continue for two or three pages. Stop. The next morning, do the same.
2. Dream Journal: Keep a journal beside your bed. Immediately upon waking, try to recall any dreams and write them down. Dreams can be ethereal or extremely vivid.
3. Gratitude Journal: Each day, list five things, or people, or places, or events, you are grateful for. Try not to repeat the same five every day.

4. Craft/Project Journal: Keep a log of a project you are working on, include photos if you wish.
5. Illustrated Journals: This is a journal that incorporates writing with drawing. You do not need to be an accomplished artist to create an illustrated journal.
6. Nature Journal: Spend time in nature and record your observations.
7. Your Cancer Journal: Keep a log of office visits, hospital stays and treatment. Include your thoughts and feelings.
8. Online journal or blog. This can be private or public. More and more cancer patients are maintaining an online journal or blog to keep family and friends updated.

The types of journals are endless. Your journal should reflect you as an individual. And you can certainly keep more than one journal. Or separate your journal into sections.

Just for fun tips: In addition to stream of consciousness writing, try writing with the hand you do not normally write with, righthanders try left, lefthanders try right.

Write down a question, pause for just a second, and then write down the very next thought that comes to you. It might be an answer. Or, try writing about yourself in third person.

9

Express

Your Creative Self

Draw. Doodle. Paint. Collage. Sculpt with clay. Work in mixed media. Take artful photographs. Pull out the trusty glue gun and get crafty. Regardless of medium, it is all art and ultimately serves the same purpose.

According to research studies, art therapy programs help cancer patients regain an identity beyond cancer, and a more hopeful outlook about the future.

Art therapy is similar to keeping a journal. Both allow for self expression. However, visual art is, for the most part, a wordless medium for those less comfortable with putting thoughts and emotions into words.

Visual art offers more benefit than moving the internal to the external world around you. An artist or crafty person will tell you there is a creative zone where time and the outside world cease to exist. The act of being creative suspends time. Stress effortlessly melts away. There are no thoughts of yesterday's cringy regrets or tomorrow's fretful future. There is the all encompassing now.

Buy yourself some art supplies and jump right in; or sign up for an art class at the community center, college or group session with an art therapist. Explore and express undiscovered and delightful dimensions of self!

10

Healing Power

of Music & Sound

"You know what music is?
God's little reminder
that there's something else besides us
in this universe; a harmonic connection
between all living beings,
everywhere, even the stars."
Robin Williams

"Hope is the thing with feathers
that perches in the soul,
and sings the tune without the words,
and never stops at all."
Emily Dickenson

As the daughter of a composer and conductor, I first learned about the power of music from stories my father shared with me.

A world traveler, he bridged communication barriers with music. Regardless of language, every human being on the planet understands, and responds to, the commonality of emotions and messages conveyed through music. My father communicated with the universal language of music, and everyone understood what was being said.

As the Robin Williams quote suggests, the power of music connects people, all living beings in our world and indeed our universe. Music gives us the opportunity to connect our inner being with our outer world as well. Becoming connected, and realizing that connection, opens a door to healing.

Since the time of the Greeks, music continues to be a recognized therapeutic tool for quieting the mind, comforting the body, lifting the spirit and soothing the soul.

Music is playing almost constantly in both the foreground and background of our daily lives. Often, we do not realize the fundamental and pervasive power of music. Music has the ability to both unite lovers and fuel revolutions. If we are feeling down, music can pull us up out of the doldrums. If we are feeling tired and unmotivated, music can energize and inspire us. If we are feeling nervous, music can calm.

And music is healing. Scientific research studies indicate a real value of music to health in lowering blood pressure, heart rate and breathing; reducing physical pain, lessening nausea, relieving mental and emotional stress; and offering an over all sense of peace and contentment for the mind, body and spirit.

The power of music in healing might prove even more profoundly significant, with the emergence of recent research findings in the field of sound therapy, actually an ancient form of healing. Music and sound therapy are both vibrational energies.

Sound therapy encompasses the use of voices in chanting; instruments such as Tibetan singing bowls, crystal bowls, bells, gongs, and drums; relaxing recordings of familiar sounds found in nature; and frequencies produced to affect a specific response in the physical body.

According to the Global Institute of Sound, the eardrum is directly connected to every organ in the body except the spleen. High frequencies activate our energy, while low frequencies calm.

A study published by Dr. Masaru Emoto, *The Effect of Intention and Prayer on Water,* is fascinating. While studying crystalline snow flake like structures formed when water freezes, Dr Emoto was able to demonstrate the power of music on these structures. Classical music created beautiful patterns while Heavy Metal created distortion. Other findings in Dr Emoto's research demonstrated the spoken word love over water created a spectacular mandala while the spoken word hate created a malformed distorted pattern.

Sacred Sound healing pioneer and founder of Sacred Sound Workshops Richard Rudis's interest in ancient Eastern Medicine vibrational philosophy and vibrational healing techniques began over 40 years ago.

Intrigued by the study results of sound on water, Rudis performed before and after blood testing to discover what might happen after a vibrational healing session. The blood testing showed remarkable results.

Some of the changes were: enhanced flow of oxygen and nutrients; red blood cells less congested; immune system stimulated; white blood cells more active, larger and brighter; and a decrease in inflammation. Rudis provides both video and photographic evidence of the results of his experiments on his website.

11

Healing Power of Humor & Laughter

"May love and laughter light your days,
and warm your heart and home.
May good and faithful friends be yours,
wherever you may roam.
May peace and plenty bless your world
with joy that long endures."

Blessing

Nothing about cancer or cancer treatment is a laughing matter, and many might find any suggestion of the humorous in any of it difficult to embrace as a "laughter is the best medicine" philosophy. Which is precisely why a daily dose of humor is so critically important.

While few will suggest laughter can cure disease, it can go a long way in easing the side effects of the seriousness of cancer, and vastly improve quality of life.

The clown doctor known as Patch Adams bases his medical profession on humor therapy. Gesundheit! Institute founder, Dr Adams believes humor and play contribute to physical and emotional health, and has traveled the world bringing humor to patients and orphans.

A famous proponent of laughter as medicine was Norman Cousins, who claims to have alleviated the pain of disease by watching Marx Brothers movies.

According to Cousins, "I made the joyous discovery that ten minutes of genuine belly laughter had an anesthetic effect and would give me at least two hours of pain-free sleep."

Over 30 years ago, laughing clubs and laughing yoga burst onto the humor therapy scene, and are thriving to this day. Typically, a group will gather and begin a few rounds of forced fake hee haw laughter. Because laughter is contagious, even repeated fake laughter will eventually lead to genuine laughter.

Laughter is compared to a mild workout and some of the health benefits of laughter are documented to include:

1. Releases endorphins, the feel good chemicals, improving mood and positive perspective
2. Decreases pain
3. Stretches and relaxes muscles used while laughing
4. Improves and strengthens immune system
5. Decreases stress, releases tension, promotes relaxation
6. Promotes a better, more restful sleep
7. Aids in digestion
8. Increases oxygen, heart rate and lung capacity
9. Lowers blood pressure
10. Lowers blood sugars
11. Promotes creativity

One of the strongest ways to bond with others is through shared laughter. Feeling connected to others is one of our basic human needs, and meeting this need supports the ability to heal.

If you feel you cannot laugh, and at times, this will be completely understandable, then smile. You will brighten your world, and the world of the person you smile at, even if it is a stranger on the street.

If you feel you cannot smile, place a pencil between your teeth and hold it there for a few minutes at a time. Holding a pencil between your teeth uses the same face muscles as a smile, and your brain does not know you are not actually smiling.

Because humor and what makes us smile and laugh is subjective, only you can know what is humorous to you. Jokes might tickle your funny bone, or watching comedy shows and movies, or ridiculous online videos. It does not matter what makes you laugh, only that you make certain to spend time laughing. Try to work in a humor break each day. YouTube can be a great resource for short humorous videos.

As a child, I was taught you can know when someone who is ill is on the road to recovery and health when they begin to laugh again. I do not know if this is true, but I do know when someone in our family was sick, and we heard them laugh for the first time, we felt confident in their returning health. Not long after, they were indeed well again. Seems this family folklore belief might end up being valid.

12

Green Medicine

"Every blade of grass has its Angel
that bends over it and whispers, Grow, grow."
Talmud

In our modern world, in our urban environment of asphalt and concrete; in our daily life of tablets and smartphones and social media; we run the risk of disconnection to our fundamental connection to the natural world and nature.

Green is the predominant color of nature. There is a reason the color green evokes deep responses of calm and inner balance. Nature reminds us of an ancient knowledge embedded in the psyche of the eternal never ending beauty and cycles of life and our intimate connection to nature. In nature, we remember who we are in relation to life and the universe outside ourselves.

In nature, we are reminded we are nature itself, in nature we are renewed to our true self.

Ideally, taking a hike in a forested area, or strolling along the banks of a river or lake is the obvious choice when we think of getting back to nature, it is not necessary to experiencing green medicine benefit. Observe the beauty surrounding you while taking a walk in your neighborhood, visiting a city park or admiring your backyard flower garden.

Keep a drawing journal or camera close at hand. Document the awe-filled every day beauty discovered.

Breath in deep the tranquility of your surroundings in the aroma of flowers and trees and all things that grow green.

This is a beautiful planet we live on with a thousand miraculous moments when we take the time to witness the delightful and the beautiful. Spend time in natural surroundings.

Bring nature into your immediate environment. Start a patio or backyard garden. From seed to mature plant, gardens are a metaphor for faith and hope for life.

July 2002

Dear Diary,

Immediately following the surgical removal of a tumor not benign, the radiologist is extolling the benefits of radiation in the treatment of cancer. The oncologist is extolling the benefits of chemotherapy. The surgeon is explaining the necessity of surgery.

The family physician is busily coordinating all the healthcare providers and treatment options.

In the dizzying and daunting immediacy of my need to make life lengthening decisions for a life threatening disease; a family friend's prescription is advising me to stay close to nature.

Connecting to the cycles and seasons of nature, to the rhythm and cadence of life in the ebb and flow of birth, death and renewal, it is easy to find my way from feeling lost to remembering the magic, meaning and purpose of being here, of being alive.

To smell the rich earth held in the hand. To hear the sound of the breeze rustling through the leaves of towering birch trees. To feel the sun beams filtering down through branches of majestic fir and cedar trees.

To watch the sight of animals living in simple agreement with the natural balance of one sunrise to sunset to sunrise to another sunset.

To taste time that does not go too fast or too slow but is eternally measured in the spaces of now; this is where the convergence of the physical and spiritual worlds meet most directly and I find myself standing in the middle with an awareness that our separation was only neglect on my part.

13

Fear In Small Doses

*"When you come to the end of your rope,
tie a knot and hang on."*

Franklin D. Roosevelt

There are two basic human emotions from which all other emotions emerge. From these two emotions we filter and define reality and react to the world around us. The two emotions are: love and fear.

Love is nourishing, sustainable, eternal, healing, grateful and life giving. Love is trust born from a core belief in a world that is generous, kind, and safe.

Fear is the opposite of love. Fear is designed to be temporary, not sustainable or eternal. However, just as much as we need love, we need fear. When facing immediate danger of any kind, fear is our internal alarm system calling us to fight or flight action. Our bodies respond by pumping high levels of adrenaline, giving us the juice to take the appropriate action needed to remove the danger or remove us from the danger. Our fear blocks out all other thoughts and is single minded in one objective: Do I fight or do I run?

The trouble we have with fear is when our fear gets stuck in default mode, overriding love and the constellation of emotions love sustains. When fear begins to filter and define our reality we are in trouble.

Fear itself becomes the danger. Because we are designed to respond to danger with fear, and fear itself becomes the danger, we are responding to fear with more fear. You can see how this can escalate and lead to feelings of unrelenting anxiety and utter hopelessness. At this point, fear can make us sick, and if we are already ill, dramatically slow the healing process.

When our body is in fear mode, and the fight or flight mechanism is activated, our system directs all our internal systems and energy to surviving the threat. This is important to understand because while this is happening, all other systems are shut down. Our immune system, and our body's ability to restore and renew and return to health, is shut down. Temporarily, this is not a problem. Sustained over time, this is a monumentally huge problem for our health.

This is why reducing fear, anxiety and stress is essential to healing.

When you are diagnosed with cancer, you suddenly find yourself in a life that is not a safe place. Cancer is an immediate danger. Initially, fear is the rational reaction. Since we cannot run away from the danger, what remains is stand and fight. However, getting from cancer diagnosis to cancer survivorship is not a temporary state of being, a here this minute gone the next minute fight.

This fight takes time and stamina. The stamina we need comes from love, not fear. We need to keep fear in perspective. Once we have decided to stand and fight, we need to resolve to put fear back in its place and return to the dominant realm of love and all the emotions of love. Fear needs to be replaced with faith that all of our fight will lead to triumph. We have responded to the danger. We no longer need fear as a call to action.

I know, putting fear in its place is easier said than done. The effective method will be as individual as the individual grappling with fear. For some, simply understanding the function and mechanism of fear is enough.

Mediation, prayer or visualization might help. Exercise might help. Joining a support group might help. Talk therapy might help.

Medications to help ease anxiety and depression might help. If you feel you might need help along these lines, be honest with your physician about your emotional struggle with fear, stress, anxiety or depression born from fear.

The message here is you are bigger than your fear and it can be put in its proper place so you can move forward and get on with your life and healing.

14

Plan for the Future

*"These things I warmly wish for you
Someone to love, some work to do,
And a guardian angel always near. "*

Blessing

Nothing says hope more than future plans. Who plans for the future unless they believe in the deepest part of their being there is a future to plan?

In this case, if you are quite uncertain about the prospect of a future for you personally, fake it till you make it.

Regardless of how you reason it out in order to do it, make plans. Make a list of all the things you would like to do in your life and all the places you would like to visit.

Make step by step plans on how to do and see all the items on your list. Take the time to make a long list.

Make your list as descriptive as possible. Add to your list as the days unfold.

Keep an open mind you will have all the time you need to accomplish every item on your list. Let your imagination play in the planning.

Plan with enthusiasm. Plan with confidence.

There is no rush or immediate need to hurry in finishing the list. You will have the time you need to see your plans through and dreams coming true.

September 2002

Dear Diary,

A cancer diagnosis is more than a curious detour that life altering experiences of life tend to represent when retrospectively measured in the spacious distance of time's wider perspective.

After learning I have cancer, I wonder how long I have left to live. One of the side effects of struggling with my own mortality is how unsure I become about tomorrow. A surly death hangs around like an obnoxious unwelcome relative on the doorstep of my mind. I have lost the certainty of hope.

I begin to wonder if hope is ever going to return. If hope will ever sit down and pull up a chair, when one day, without announcement, hope is back.

Hope sashays into the room, throws all the curtains open, fills the room with light, settles in and flashes its brilliant smile of reassurance. I am not about to quarrel about the abandonment. I am far too ecstatic at the return of hope to quibble over departure and arrival times.

We are, hope and I, busily back to making plans.

15

Forgiveness & Letting Go

"Come out of the circle of time,
and into the circle of love. "
Rumi

"May God grant you always a sunbeam
to warm you,
a moonbeam to charm you,
a sheltering angel, so nothing can harm you."
Blessing

Forgiveness: How does anyone forgive the deliberately harmful, the unthinkable, the unforgivable?

Letting go: Why does anyone feel it is right or just to walk away from another person's wrongdoing, to let them off the hook?

Because it benefits you, the recipient of, or witness to, the original harm. Although it sounds counter intuitive, forgiveness and letting go have nothing to do with allowing the other person to get away without answering for their horrible actions and everything to do with freeing you from unnecessary torment.

You might have a monumental struggle with forgiveness and letting go, most decent people do. You might feel, if you do not remember, who will? If you do not hold the wrongdoer accountable, even if only in your mind, who will? Understandable.

The problem is the brain operates in complex, and at times, perplexing ways. When it comes to memory, the brain does not seem to differentiate the event you are remembering as something that happened in the past to something that is happening now.

For the brain, the memory you are remembering is happening now. Again. And each time you remember it. Your physical body will react as if the memory is happening now, even if it is something that happened years ago.

Each time you re-live the memory, the event is harming you again, and again, and again.

The unfortunate ultimate truth is, while you are ruminating in pain, anger, hate, and judgment, the object of your unforgiveness is often blithely living their life without a care in the world for what you remember.

In holding on to the memory of the unforgivable, the only person who continues to be harmed by the harm is you.

From every tiny tear of the heart to knockout punches to the soul, all the deep down inside loneliness, memories of abandonment, coldness, resentment, anger, grudges, or physical and emotional injury, how does anyone move on? I will share with you how I was successfully able to forgive and let go.

Write letters, long letters, to each person you had a difficult relationship with and to anyone who has caused you irreparable harm.

Write and write and write until you have nothing else to say, and say it all.

Then ceremonially build a fire in the wood stove or fireplace or at the next campfire and watch each letter burn until it is pure ash. Until it is gone. Make a conscious decision to turn and walk away.

Forgiveness is not about letting the other person go scot free or minimizing the harm they caused. Forgiveness is ending the power of the other person's original harm to harm you again and again by remembering the harm. By letting go, you are not allowing it another minute of thought or feeling.

You have a right to have your say, and you might not have ever exercised this right.

Writing letters is a safe and effective means of having your say. Burning the letters to ash is letting go. With letting go, you create more room for healing and free yourself from any additional harm.

Nothing, and I mean nothing, that happened in all of your yesterdays matter today. Today is all that matters. This is your reality, you have the power to define it rather than allowing anyone else define your reality for you.

You are standing in the middle of a warm, loving, giving, beautiful life. Your life.

"May you always have

Walls for the winds

A roof for the rain

Tea beside the fire

Laughter to cheer you

Those you love near you

And all your heart might desire."

Blessing

16

You are Not Alone

*"There are only two ways to live your life.
One is as though nothing is a miracle.
The other is as if everything is."*

Albert Einstein

Not talking religion, unless you are religiously inclined. Not talking specific spirituality, if you are grounded in more pragmatic scientific sensibilities.

I am talking about the darkest night of the soul and the benefit of not feeling alone. Even if you do not believe in guardian angels, or God, or a divine operating universal intelligence of any kind, it is important you feel connected to something larger than yourself. Something that is benevolent, compassionate and caring.

If you belong to a group or community where you are loved, completely and unconditionally loved, have always been cared for and loved beyond measure, then you are extremely fortunate and blessed.

However, if there are times you might not have felt you were cared for and loved unconditionally; if there were times when you questioned whether there is a purpose and meaning to your individual life; I am suggesting you were, are now and will always be cared for, supported and believed in and loved by that something that is bigger than yourself.

You were never, and are not now, and never will be, alone. You are not separate. No one is, nothing is, as even science proves. We are all interconnected in this field of energy.

What you choose to call it is up to you, but it exists and you exist within it.

Even if you need to suspend your current beliefs that there are no guardian angels, or God, or a divine operating universal intelligence of any kind, accept there might be more to life than meets the eye and search for a concept in this paradigm most comfortable for you.

Before you go to bed at night, repeat the thought you live in a kind, loving, giving, generous, safe world until you drift off to sleep. Feel genuinely grateful as you think this thought.

When you wake in the morning, before you get out of bed, start the day by telling yourself you will meet with kindness and generosity as you move through a safe world.

As I move through my day, I imagine the very air around me is the energy field of love, and each time I inhale, I am inhaling the energy of love. This love fills every cell of my body.

Hold fast that love, providence and grace are with you always in all ways and you will discover the miraculous expansion of connection your constant companion.

17

Obligation in Giving Back

*"When you are inspired by some great purpose,
some extraordinary project,
all of your thoughts break their bonds, your mind
transcends limitations,
your consciousness expands in every direction
and you find yourself in a new
great and wonderful world. Dormant forces,
faculties and talents become alive,
and you discover yourself
to be a greater person by far
than you ever dreamed yourself to be."*

Patanjali

*"To those whom much is given,
much is required."*
Luke 12:48

I cannot name them by name or hold the image of their faces in my mind, because I do not know their names and I have not seen their faces.

I do carry each of them in my grateful heart for each morning that I wake again. The research renegades and the rebels of convention, the pioneers exploring unmapped microscopic territories and the altruistic money movers and policy makers.

Most of all, I am indebted to the women who volunteered for experimental treatments that might or might not have helped them to live longer, but led to the current treatments that help me live longer.

Some cancer survivors might not be comfortable sharing their story in oral or written form, or have the celebrity or motivation to start a cancer survivor organization, and that is more than acceptable.

There are any number of ways to give back for the ultimate gift of more life given. The importance is assessing your talents and abilities in finding a way to give back to all those who came before you and all who will come after you.

It is our obligation as a cancer survivors.

October 2002

Dear Diary,

According to the official count, 38,000 people participated in the Susan G. Komen Breast Cancer Race For The Cure today. The 5K Co-Ed Walk officially begins at 9:30 am. The shoulder to shoulder lines of walkers stretches back for many city blocks, and it takes us 20 minutes from where we stand in line to pass under the starting arch.

We are in a sea of people in pink: survivors wearing pink hats and shirts; survivor family and friends wearing 12 inch pink square signs pinned to the back of their clothing to honor someone surviving breast cancer or someone lost to breast cancer.

Ahead of us, people crossing the Burnside Bridge span all six lanes. As many people are walking behind us as are walking before us, participants visually reaching the horizon in both directions. We are each part of something bigger than the self and if the healing power of heaven can be pulled down to touch the earth we are walking on, surely it is now.

There are bagpipes and drumming as we walk. Cheering and bottled water. Those wearing pink hats are handed a rose as they cross the finish line.

I am the only one wearing a pink hat on the shuttle bus ride back to the east side of Portland, when a fellow rider asks why I walk in the Race For The Cure.

In gratitude, I walk for all the women who walked before me and because of them I am still here. In support, I walk for all the women who will walk after me, who do not know they will be walking in the race, who will be told this year or the next year they have breast cancer.

I walk in hope, so when the day comes, if it does, and they tell me my cancer is back, maybe the walking done today will make a difference when a difference is most needed.

But most of all, I walk for the little girl who walks in the race today, with the 12 inch pink square pinned to the back of her sweatshirt that reads — In Memory Of ... My Mom.

The rain has threatened to fall all day and does not during the charity event. As we are chatting, the rain begins to stream down the shuttle bus windows, softly at first, then more intensely. It is as if the world weeps for the losses that come too soon and should not have come at all for the now motherless and fatherless children and still the losses happen when all we can do is still not enough. We will keep showing up, we will keep trying, we will not give up.

18

Write Love Letters

"Angels around us
angels beside us
angels within us
Angels are watching over you
when times are good or stressed
Their wings wrap gently around you
Whispering you are loved and blessed."

Blessing

"We can do no great things,
only small things with great love."

Mother Teresa

Having been on both sides of the cancer diagnosis fence, of being diagnosed with cancer and as a family member of someone diagnosed with cancer, I can say with authenticity of experience it is easier to be the cancer patient. At least as a cancer patient, you are engaged in the process, busily tromping and trudging through the treatments for cancer and navigating the aftercare of cancer survivorship.

On an emotional and physical stress level, a cancer diagnosis affects family and friends in the same devastating way it does for the loved one diagnosed with cancer. Since everyone and everything is focused on the patient, the support, resources and attention to the needs of family and friends can be incidental to nonexistent.

While dealing with the trauma of cancer as much as the patient, family and friends often get lost in the shuffle. If you are to ask, they will have it no other way. They will tell you they do not need anything, other than, "please help, please save my loved one from the dreadful disease".

Family and friends of a cancer patient are suffering. Nothing feels more hopeless than standing on the side lines watching someone you love struggle through the shock of a cancer diagnosis and different stages of cancer treatment and knowing there is little, if anything, you can do to affect the circumstance or outcome.

Family and friends live in a helpless hopeless state of constant fear; who feel they can do nothing more than watch; do nothing more than hold their loved one's hand as they hold their own fearful breath; do nothing more than whisper prayers and petitions to the intelligence of this universe for mercy and grace for their loved one facing a fight for life; who would make bargains of any kind to gain a healthy long life for their loved one if only they knew who or what to strike that bargain.

One of the aspects of cancer treatment for the cancer patient is the down time of recuperation and recovery.

During this time, write love letters to your family and friends. In the form of handwritten letters or poems, let them know the love, courage, strength, and unending prayer they express on your behalf nourishes your spirit, strengthens your determined will, comforts your discomfort and inspires your reach for tomorrow. And that no matter what happens, their love made life so beautifully bearable in even the worst moments of this journey.

19

Create a Healing Shrine

"May God heal you, body and soul.
May your pain cease.
May your strength increase.
May your fears be released.
May blessings, love and joy surround you. Amen."
Prayer

"El na refa na lah."
Please God, bring healing.
Prayer

"May the blessing of light be on you, light without
and light within."

Blessing

A healing shrine can reside on a bookshelf, end table, in the corner of a room, or if space allows, and entire room. A healing shrine can reside outside, in a covered space to protect against the elements. Basically, chose an area where the healing shrine will not be disturbed, where there is no need to move it, or worse yet, clutter it with any objects not a part it.

The purpose of a healing shrine is creating a space, a place, an environment for that which inspires and sustains us, the tranquility of peace and nurturance of love. A place of respite and renewal where we find balance in quiet connection to our inner self and to the something bigger than the self.

Because a healing shrine is as personal as the person creating it, there are no rules as to how it should be designed or the objects chosen for it. Choose objects that speak to your heart. To start you thinking about your healing shrine, I will share some objects I placed in mine:

A box containing inspirational quotes, prayers and stories of healing; photos of my loved ones, both family and friends; rocks and other momentos my children would give me as a gift on visits to the ocean or a walk by the river; a crystal beaded necklace given to me as a gift; a rose scented candle given to me as a gift. The color theme of my healing shrine is blue and green; the colors of sky and all that grows on earth.

20

Avoid Toxic People

*"May joy and peace surround you,
contentment latch your door,
and happiness be with you now
and bless you evermore!"*
Blessing

*"May God give you
For every storm, a rainbow,
For every tear, a smile,
For every care, a promise,
And a blessing in each trial.
For every problem life sends,
A faithful friend to share,
For every sigh, a sweet song,
And an answer for each prayer."*
Blessing

We all have them in our life, and we all know who they are, and we all put up with them.

Even though no one is all good or all bad, and someone who is toxic for you might be absolutely adorable to someone else; this is not so much a judgment call, as it is being clear on who affirms life and who does not – for you.

Toxic people are the people, who on the surface might appear nice, but whenever we spend time with them, we leave the experience feeling this vague persistent negativity about ourselves or life. Some times, they do not even put the effort into appearing nice to disguise the negativity. These people can be family members, coworkers, friends or the grocery checker at the local market.

If you cannot avoid these people, limit your exposure as much as possible. Try to keep your interactions on a polite and shallow level. Try not to listen too intently to their conversations. Try not to internalize any of their messages.

When you must spend time with them, mentally visualize a protective bubble surrounding you and protecting you from their toxicity. Most importantly, make certain you create a network of people in your life who inspire you, who make you laugh, who remind you of all kindness, beauty and love of life.

21

Fill Your Life With Beauty

*"Today,
like every other day,
we wake up empty and frightened.
Don't open the door to the study
and begin reading.*

*Let the beauty we love be what we do.
There are hundreds of ways
to kneel and kiss the ground."*

Rumi

You can tell much about how you think and how you feel by observing the state of your habitat, your home. Our external surroundings will both impress and reflect our internal state of being. Creating a beautiful environment contributes to a healing environment.

But first, before we discuss bringing beauty into your surroundings, let's talk about clutter creep, and how it adversely affects health.

Clutter happens incrementally at first, then without noticing, there is a drawer, closet, desktop, bookcase, spare room, or garage crowded and overflowing with, well, all manner of things.

For example, I can tell I have some level of difficulty focusing on one thing at a time by the disarray of stacks of papers and books on my desk. Which in turn leads to the realization I might be creating more underlying stress for myself than I realize or need to, this disorganized disarray of reflected thinking and being. I can tell you I might not be someone who deals with all my issues as they arise, because I have junk drawers in more than one room and a closet in serious and chronic need of organizing. When I do decide to clear the clutter, to organize my space, I get clearer and less stressed, and life seems easier and lighter for both my mind and emotions.

I bring up the dreaded clutter creep conversation because in order to fill your life with beauty, to create an environment of calm and beauty for the mind, heart and spirit, it is far better to start with a space that is clear of clutter. Clutter will compete and potentially negate efforts at bringing lasting beauty into your surroundings.

A few tips on decluttering clutter creep. Start small. Looking at the entirety of the project can feel daunting. For example, do one junk drawer a day. One bookshelf, one corner of a room, one section of your desk.

Now, to creating a beautiful environment for every day living. Fill your home with colors you love, aromas you adore, art prints and books that move your soul. Buy yourself fresh cut flowers each week. Decorate your home by season.

For example, my dining room centerpiece reflects the season. In fall, I walk and gather large fallen dried maple leaves, adding gourds and decorative pumpkins. In winter, pine cones, candles and evergreen branches. In spring, decorative eggs; in summer, bowls of fresh seasonal fruits.

For the bath, fill a basket with fragrant soaps, lotions and oils; plush washcloths and loofahs,

Epsom bath salts stored into a decorative container. Invest in luxurious thick quality made towels. Make your bed as comfortable as possible. Add a foam topper, invest in the softest sheets and comfiest comforters possible. Buy new pillows. You are so worth it.

Turn the pages of home decor, craft and holiday theme magazines or browse the internet for decorating ideas to beautify your surroundings. Stop at garage sales; visit secondhand, thrift and antique stores to recreate ideas that appeal to you. Creating beauty in your home and expressing your individual tastes does not require huge expense.

Fill your life with organizations you believe in and people you hold most dear. The beauty you choose to surround yourself with and the meaningful ways you choose to spend your time will affect and reflect your inner state of being.

Beauty is more than an aesthetically pleasing luxury. Beauty, in all its forms, is essential as an expression of the optimistic goodness of, and appreciation for life.

Fill your life with beauty and meaning where hope and healing has the optimum chance to flourish. Honor yourself at all times and celebrate your life continuously in ways small and large.

22

Expect To Be a Survivor

As a cancer patient, one of the first questions you will feel compelled to ask involves your odds of surviving cancer. We want to know the answer, and simultaneously, we fear what the answer holds for us.

Each cancer is different, and the body of statistical evidence offers generalized information of percentages and odds for your specific cancer. Take this information with a grain of salt. Statistics mean absolutely nothing to the individual outcomes for the patient diagnosed with cancer. Living and dying are very personal, individualistic and subjective issues.

There are stories of people who are told they have three months to live and go on to live 15 or more additional years. There are people who are told they have a 95 percent chance of easily surviving cancer for five years and sadly, do not live five more years.

If the protocols for treatment are roughly the same for the same type of cancer, what is it that keeps someone who is not expected to live three more months still alive 15 years later?

When the person given the glowing prediction they will live another five years, probably 10 years, possibly 20 years, passes so much sooner than the statistics suggest?

There are better questions than what the cancer survival odds are as predicted by statisticians, and they are:

What does the person, who defied the odds, know that I might not know? What did they do to make statistics of interest and relevance to no one other than statisticians?

"There are more things in heaven and earth, Horatio, than are dreamt of in your philosophy."
Shakespeare

I want to understand the more things in heaven and earth than I had dreamt of up to now. Most of what I learned, in one form or the other, is in this book.

Before the diagnosis of cancer, I did not know the time and date of my death. I still do not know. You do not know the time and date of your death. No one does, whether they have been diagnosed with a life threatening disease or not. We are not required to accept anyone knows with certainty.

Begin each day with every expectation you will live as a long term cancer survivor. Each day you wake up, you are right in your expectations for living. Be glad. Be thankful.

Each day you wake up, after giving thanks for another new day, realize you might be one day closer to that time when research comes up with a treatment that ends the need for more treatment. New breakthrough advances in treatment are being announced with amazing regularity. Who knows what is just around the corner.

Each day you wake up, and after giving thanks for another new day, tell yourself, tell the universe, you plan on sticking around so you won't miss the announcement.

Each day you wake up, after giving thanks for another new day, plan your life as if you have a thousand years to live and live each day as if it is the only one that ever happens.

Each cancer diagnosis needs to include a philosophy of pronoia disclaimer, as explained by Pronoia author Rob Brezsny:

"Pronoia.
The opposite of paranoia.

Pronoia is defined as the sneaking suspicion
that the whole world is conspiring
to shower you with blessings."

Especially for healing: expect blessings.

You Are Not Cancer

Cancer happened to you, it is not who you are, it does not define you. You are not cancer.

In fact, I will go as far as to say, except for the medical appointments you need to keep and related business you need to attend to, do not give cancer much thought at all. Go on living your life to the fullest, and focus on the beauty, love and meaning of life.

Bad things happen to very good people. You are a good person and the bad thing that is happening to you is cancer. Cancer is an event, not an identity.

Identify with the survivors, not the cancer. Today, there are many cancer survivors and there is every reason for you to believe you will survive cancer and thrive as a cancer survivor too. Even stage four cancer patients, the stage where cure is no longer considered a viable option, are living longer almost to the point where stage four treatments resemble treatment for long term chronic diseases.

Live in the abundance and beauty and love and meaning of now. Make peace with life and find the place within yourself where you discover all that you are meant to express in this world, and then fearlessly give all that you are to each day, and accept with gratitude and love all that life has to offer.

Live as big as you can, expanding yourself to fill every space of your life, for every minute of every day you are given this gift of life. In quiet ways. In loud ways. In all ways. On your own terms. Set out to live each day fully, and make each day worth a lifetime.

With love, I wrote this guide for you.

"May the road rise up to meet you.

May the wind be always at your back.

May the rain fall soft upon your fields.
And, until we meet again,

may God hold you in the palm of His hand."

Blessing

and always remember this:

We are our stories.
What story are you choosing to tell?

An Afterword ... or two

With little understanding or explanation, spontaneous remission happens. To date it is considered a rare phenomenon. But how rare an occurrence, is up for some debate. Few individuals or organizations attempt to understand spontaneous remission. Because it appears to us as a mystery, spontaneous remission might actually go underreported. What can we say, what do we usually say, about a mystery, other than to give a who knows shrug of the shoulders and carry on, remaining in the framework of what we do understand; the logical, the explainable, the predictable.

Fortunate for all of us, there lives still, a pioneering spirit, in the minds and hearts of both men and women of science and organizations who make it their mission to understand the mysteries. In addition to the men and women mentioned throughout this guide, I will introduce you to three more forward thinking men of science, Dr Bernard "Bernie" Siegel, Dr Bruce Lipton and Gregg Braden; and one organization, The Institute of Noetic Sciences (IONS).

IONS states while spontaneous remission is uncommon, the number of reported cases is on the rise. The more cases reported, the closer to discovering a common thread, if there is one. If it happens once, then more than once, it becomes more than a fleeting possibility of the same event happening again and again and again. Our current dilemma is understanding how and why spontaneous remission can happen at all.

IONS defines spontaneous remission as follows:

"spontaneous remission is the disappearance, complete or incomplete, of a disease or cancer without medical treatment or treatment that is considered inadequate to produce the resulting difference of disease symptoms or tumor".

In the 1990's, IONS launched the Remission Project. The culmination of that project led to the largest database of medically reported cases of spontaneous remission in the world, with more than 3,500 references from more than 800 journals in 20 languages. Compiled by Caryle Hirschberg and Brendan O'Regan, Spontaneous Remission: An Annotated Bibliography is available as a free 713-page pdf download through the IONS website.

There are a growing number of new voices bridging science and spirituality, bringing a new understanding of integrative mind body healing and a shift in paradigm for achieving and maintaining optimum health.

One of the better-known leaders in epigenetics is stem cell biologist and medical school professor Dr Bruce Lipton. Briefly, epigenetics is the study of gene function not explained by changes in DNA sequence, with epi meaning on top of, outside of, and genetics meaning the study of genes.

According to Dr Lipton,

"Experiments reveal that the cell membrane, the outer layer of the cell, is the organic equivalent of a computer chip, and the cell's equivalent of a brain. Although this view conflicts with the widely held scientific dogma that genes control behavior, papers by other researchers have validated my thinking".

And while traditional cell biology focuses on the physical molecules that control biology, Dr Lipton's interest in the principles of quantum physics to the field of cellular biology and work focuses on the mechanisms through which energy in the form of beliefs can affect our biology and genetic code.

This goes far beyond the power of positive or negative thinking, which on its own produces little effect. In fact, thoughts on their own are almost completely ineffective if not connected and cemented to a corresponding emotion. Both thought and emotion combined create a belief.

Most of our beliefs are formed early in life, long before most of us remember, and embedded in our subconscious. And according to Dr Lipton, 95 percent of our beliefs reside in the subconscious.

The original foundation of our belief system was created by the dominant figures in our earliest formative years when we had little say and choice in the matter. It hardly seems possible, but what we think we believe in our adult years (conscious) and what our true beliefs are (subconscious) can be dramatically at odds with the other.

Which is why, change can seem so difficult and even insurmountable. If you are making a conscious choice to change an aspect of yourself or your life, but your subconscious has a belief that opposes the conscious change choice, the subconscious, the 95 percent of your belief system, will be completely unfazed by your effort.

Becoming aware of this, we can tap into and reprogram our subconscious beliefs to match our conscious thought. Create a coherent belief system of our choosing; more in line with the vision we wish to hold for our life, including our health.

Gregg Braden is a computer geologist drawn to the study of ancient texts and how that wisdom can be brought forward and interpreted and integrated with what we know in modern science. Some of what we understand today the ancients spoke of and wrote down in sacred texts, only in a much different language and from a much different perspective.

According to Braden,

"In 1944, Max Planck, the father of quantum theory, stated there is a "matrix" of energy providing the blueprint for our physical world. The experimental proof that Planck's matrix is real, provides the missing link bridging our spiritual experiences of imagination, prayer and beliefs with the miracles we see in the world around us. Through the connection that joins all things, scientists have shown the "stuff" the universe is made of – waves and particles of energy – responds and conforms to the expectations and judgments and beliefs we create about our world. "

The title of Dr Bernard "Bernie" Siegel's first book Love Medicine and Miracles, his following book Peace, Love & Healing and his latest book A Book Of Miracles – Inspiring True Stories of Healing, Gratitude and Love tell you much about the mind, heart and wisdom of a man of medicine whose work is raising awareness of the mind body connection for both the medical profession and patients.

In 1978, Bernie established Exceptional Cancer Patients, EcaP, an art therapy and humor approach Bernie calls Carefrontation where patients interpret their drawings, dreams and recognize symbols to express and understand these messages for healing.

According to Bernie,

"In the next decade, the roles of consciousness, spirituality, non-local healing, body memory and heart energy will be explored more intensively as scientific subjects".

As a final thought for the reader of this guide; cancer treatment, and life after cancer, can be financially expensive. Even with insurance, there are expenses.

Almost every idea of the 22 ideas presented in this guide can be followed without any (or minimal) financial cost or researched without financial cost through simple searches on the internet – through websites, blogs or viewing YouTube videos.

In addition, refer to the online resources listed at the end of this guide. Lastly, before purchasing a book, CD, or movie, check your local library.

Resources

(mentioned in this guide)

National Center for Complementary and Alternative Medicine (NCCAM)

http://nccam.nih.gov/health/atoz.htm

NCCAM is the leading US government agency for scientific research on complementary, alternative and integrative medicine. Extensive database on alternative therapies including Herbs at a Glance.

American Institute of Cancer Research (AICR)

www.aicr.org

For 30 years, AICR has conducted nutrition, diet, physical activity, cancer prevention, treatment and survival research for the purposes of establishing dietary links to cancer and cancer prevention. Information and resources include AICR's Foods That Fight Cancer

Patch Adams, The Gesundheit! Institute

www.patchadams.org

Medical doctor, clown and social activist Patch Adams believes laughter, joy and creativity is an integral part of the healing process. The Gesundheit! Institute serves as a model for holistic medical care based on the belief the health of the individual, family, society and world cannot be separated.

Richard Rudis, Sacred Sound Gong Bath

www.sacredsoundgongbath.com

American practitioner of Vajrayana School of Tibetan Buddhism Richard Rudis is a long time pilgrim of sacred sites and teaching across Asia. He teaches Buddhist Dharma and conducts Vibrational Sound Healing Workshops using traditional Himalayan instruments.

To view results of before and after blood testing video and photos to discover what happened after a vibrational healing session, visit this page:

www.sacredsoundgongbath.com/blood-testing.html

Global Institute of Sound & Consciousness
www.soundhealingcenter.com

An extensive educational website on sound therapy and research projects on physiological, metabolic, voice, morphogenetic, brainwave, emotion and etheric frequencies.

Dr Bernie Siegel, Love Medicine & Miracles

www.berniesiegelmd.com

Bestselling author of 11 books, Bernie, whose first is Love, Medicine & Miracles and latest A Book Of Miracles: Inspiring Stories of Healing, Gratitude and Love is an advocate for patient empowerment, mind body connection in healing, and "humanizing" medical practices.

Dr Bruce Lipton

www.brucelipton.com

Dr Bruce Lipton's official website.

Gregg Braden

www.greggbraden.com

Gregg Braden's official website.

Brian Weiss

www.brianweiss.com

Chairman Emeritus of Psychiatry at Mount Sinai Medical Center in Miami, psychotherapist and best selling author of Many Lives, Many Masters Dr Brian Weiss is best known for past life regressions using guided meditation. If past life regression is not of interest, a remarkably effective guided meditation by Dr Weiss for relaxation is Meditation: Achieving Inner Peace and Tranquility in Your Life.

Jon Kabat-Zinn

www.mindfulnesscds.com

Professor of Medicine Emeritus at University of Massachusetts Medical School and founder of the Mindful Based Stress Reduction Clinic, Jon Kabat-Zinn is considered one of the leading authorities in mindfulness and is the author of books and guided mindfulness meditations.

Early research focused on the mind body connection for healing and mindfulness meditation training for, among other groups, cancer patients.

Belleruth Naperstek

www.healthjourneys.com

Psychotherapist Belleruth Naperstek offers a catalog of guided meditation and guided imagery CDs for cancer patients, including:

Meditations for Chemotherapy, Promote Successful Surgery, Ease Pain, Healthful Sleep, Fight Cancer, Relieve Stress and General Wellness.

Patrick Murphy

www.sterlingheart.com

Drawing on their experience as hospice volunteers, Sterling Heart founders, Sandi Kimmel and Patrick Murphy, created the HEART WIDE OPEN - Self-Care for Caregivers handbook of techniques designed to aid everyone who has ever cared for anyone else.

Sandi Kimmel

www.sandikimmel.com

Singer songwriter, music healer and inspirational workshop leader of ancient wisdom, positive messages and sing out-loud songs.

The Institute of Noetic Sciences (IONS)

http://noetic.org/library/publication-bibliographies/spontaneous-remission-annotated-bibliography/

Spontaneous Remission: An Annotated Bibliography (713-page pdf download) is available at no cost through the url listed above.

For continuing inspiration, information and resources in the fields of alternative therapies, integrative treatments and mind body medicine, you are welcome to visit:

www.hopeandhealing.com